A Journal of Care

I0416298

Journal For: _____

Journal Covers: _____ *thru* _____
(Journal Covers Only One Month)

By: Richard Kreis
A Certified Caregiving Consultant

Cover Photograph and Editing
By: Trish Hughes Kreis

A QUICK NOTE FROM THE AUTHOR

This book could not have happened without the health issues my mother, brother-in-law and I have gone through over the years. With the help of my wife, doctors, nurses, emergency room staff and emergency medical technicians and with both of us being caregivers to loved ones we've learned the simplest way to get all of your loved one's information into the medical staff's hands when needed.

Thanks to everyone for helping me to streamline this booklet and to all the caregivers out there. Thank you for all that you do; you do more than you realize.

© 2016 iCare Consulting and Richard Kreis

ISBN 978-1-365-17338-7

Published by: iCare Consulting and Richard Kreis, Sacramento, Ca.

"Pain Without Humor is Just Painful"

~ Richard Kreis

TABLE OF CONTENTS

ACKNOWLEDGEMENTS

This book would never have come to be without my loving wife, Trish, my mother (who without her teachings I would not be who I am today) and Robert, my most excellent brother-in-law, and the many trips we have made to various emergency rooms, doctors, surgery centers and therapists offices of all kinds over the past many years.

I do have to add a special thank you to all the families and patients we have met or been roommates with while in the various hospitals and again to all the medical and hospital personnel we have met and to all those I may have forgotten to mention. To all those we have spoken to, interacted with, complained to and even laughed with: without all of you our journeys would not have been near as pleasant.

Thank you all for your assistance, time, drive and dedication which I'm sure at times feels unrewarding. My mom loves the saying,

"It is What It Is"

Yet, all of you made "It" so much easier. Thank you.

A very special thank you to Gincy, Kathy, Pegi and Trish for allowing me to work with them on,"365 Caregiving Tips: Practical Tips from Everyday Caregivers." Which you will find some of those tips are listed in here. It is their friendship and honesty that has helped me realize that I could write this book.

Thank you all,

Richard Kreis

"Every day I wake up is going to a great day."

~ Richard Kreis

INTRODUCTION

When you go to any doctor's appointment, lab work, physical therapy or any other medical office, go in with a list of questions and ask them. I know I'm not a doctor and I don't have a Ph.D. after my name, yet my background includes caring for my chronic back condition for 23 plus years, caring for my mother after several strokes about 6-8 years ago and then after her major lung surgery, a dual heart valve replacement a few years later, a fall causing a spiral break of her femur causing her to be stationary for almost nine months and all her follow up care since then. I also provide care along with my wife for my brother-in-law who has epilepsy and who has lived with us for almost four years now. You could say that I have a Ph.D. in On the Job Medical Aid Assistant if that were a position.

As you are filling in these pages and you think of questions you may have for your doctor as you think of them add them to a list just don't wait until the last minute, I guarantee you will forget some of them if you wait. Make sure your medication list(s) are up to date. Not one of the hundreds of appointments we have gone to over the past 6-8 years has the various hospitals ever been correct with mom's current medications and they prescribed them! (See medication list page). This ensures you don't receive medications that interact with others you are taking, medications get refilled at the right time and every doctor you see in on the same page with all the others.

When the doctor is telling you what he thinks the issue is or what treatment he/she is suggesting and you don't quite understand what they mean, "Ask Questions," have them write the information down. New medication(s), write it down. Body part being affected and name is issue, write it down. Then when you get home you will have the correct information and spelling to do a search on the internet. Make sure you fully understand the situation prior to saying yes to anything. Just because they have "Dr." in their name does not mean you can't talk to them or ask questions. Most doctors appreciate the patient who asks questions. It shows you're involved with your health.

Live Well,
Richard Kreis

MEDICAL INFORMATION

DATE: _____ AGE: _____

NAME: _____

LISTS OF CONTACTS

PRIMARY CONTACT: _____
RELATIONSHIP TO YOU: MOTHER, FATHER, SPOUSE, SIBLING, OTHER
ADDRESS: _____
CITY: _____ STATE: _____ ZIP: _____

SECONDARY CONTACT: _____
RELATIONSHIP TO YOU: MOTHER, FATHER, SPOUSE, SIBLING, OTHER
ADDRESS: _____
CITY: _____ STATE: _____ ZIP: _____

INSURANCE INFORMATION

PRIMARY INSURANCE: _____
POLICY NUMBER: _____ GROUP #: _____
CONTACT NAME: _____
PHONE #: _____ FAX #: _____
EMAIL: _____

SECONDARY INSURANCE: _____
POLICY NUMBER: _____ GROUP #: _____
CONTACT NAME: _____
PHONE #: _____ FAX #: _____
EMAIL: _____

ADDITIONAL INSURANCE: _____
POLICY NUMBER: _____ GROUP #: _____
CONTACT NAME: _____
PHONE #: _____ FAX #: _____
EMAIL: _____

MEDICAL CONTACTS

PRIMARY PHYSICAN: _____
SPECIALITY: _____
PHONE #: _____ FAX #: _____
EMAIL: _____

SPECIALIST #1: _____
SPECIALITY: _____
PHONE #: _____ FAX #: _____
EMAIL: _____

SPECIALIST #2: _____
SPECIALITY: _____
PHONE #: _____ FAX #: _____
EMAIL: _____

SPECIALIST #3: _____
SPECIALITY: _____
PHONE #: _____ FAX #: _____
EMAIL: _____

SPECIALIST #4: _____
SPECIALITY: _____
PHONE#: _____ FAX #: _____
EMAIL: _____

THERAPIST: _____
SPECIALITY: _____
PHONE#: _____ FAX#: _____
EMAIL: _____

OTHER: _____
SPECIALITY: _____
PHONE #: _____ FAX#: _____
EMAIL: _____

PHARMACY CONTACTS

PHARMACY #1: _____

ADDRESS: _____

CITY: _____ STATE: _____ ZIP: _____

PHARMACY #2: _____

ADDRESS: _____

CITY: _____ STATE: _____ ZIP: _____

"The pain you feel today will be the strength you feel tomorrow"

~ Unknown

MISCELLANEOUS INFORMATION

_____

_____

_____

_____

_____

_____

_____

_____

_____

_____

_____

_____

_____

_____

_____

CURRENT MEDICAL CONDITION(S)

AS OF: _____/_____/_____

__PRIMARY CONDITION:__ _____

_____

_____

PAIN LEVEL: _____ HOW LONG: _____ WORST TIME OF DAY: _____

SYMPTOMS:

_____

_____

_____

__SECONDARY CONDITION:__

_____

_____

_____

PAIN LEVEL: _____ HOW LONG: _____ WORST TIME OF DAY: _____

SYMPTOMS:

_____

_____

_____

__ADDITIONAL CONDITIONS:__

_____

_____

_____

PAIN LEVEL: _____ HOW LONG: _____ WORST TIME OF DAY: _____

SYMPTOMS:

_____

_____

_____

"For every challenge encountered there is opportunity for growth."

~ Unknown

TIPS FOR MEDICATIONS AND SUPPLEMENTS

- *Enter medications and supplements alphabetically on lists.*

- ***Tip #92*** "Using a permanent marker, write the refill date on top of the bottle cap. With one glance you can see when it is time for a refill." *

- ***Tip #47*** "Keep a daily log making note of daily activities, mood and physical problems." *

- ***Tip #48*** *"Take the log to doctor appointments as it may help explain a new behavior or health issue." **

- *Both the caregiver and patient should carry a current medication list in case of an emergency.*

- *A medication list should include all medications & supplements.*

- ***Tip #96*** *Program the pharmacy's phone number into your phone. You will have the number when you need it to ask a question about a prescription, need to reorder a medication or in case of an emergency.*

These tips are excerpts from:
"365 Caregiving Tips: Practical Tips from Everyday Caregivers."

CURRENT MEDICATIONS

MEDICATION	DOSAGE	# PER DAY	AM/PM

1. _____

2. _____

3. _____

4. _____

5. _____

6. _____

7. _____

8. _____

9. _____

10. _____

11. _____

12. _____

13. _____

14. _____

15. _____

NOTE: *List as much information here as possible*

"Every day is an Excellent Day"

~ Robert Wright

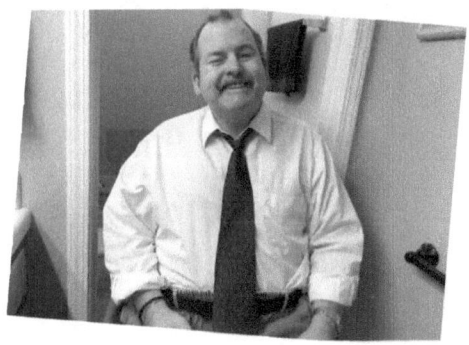

CURRENT SUPPLEMENTS

SUPPLEMENT	DOSAGE	# PER DAY	AM/PM

1. _____
2. _____
3. _____
4. _____
5. _____
6. _____
7. _____
8. _____
9. _____
10. _____

NOTE: Many supplements have been known to cause side effects with prescription medications, please list "_All Supplements_" you are taking.

ALLERGIES AND THEIR SIDE EFFECTS

ALLERGY	SIDE EFFECT

1. _____
2. _____
3. _____
4. _____
5. _____
6. _____
7. _____
8. _____
9. _____
10. _____

PREVIOUS SURGERIES OR PROCEDURES WITH DATES

	SURGERY	DATES

1. _____

2. _____

3. _____

4. _____

5. _____

6. _____

7. _____

8. _____

9. _____

10. _____

WEBSITES OR BLOG YOU FOLLOW REGARDING CONDITIONS

1. _____

2. _____

3. _____

4. _____

5. _____

6. _____

7. _____

8. _____

9. _____

10. _____

WHAT ARE YOUR CURRENT & LONG TERM GOALS?

```
|-----|-----|-----|-----|-----|-----|-----|-----|-----|-----|
  0    1    2    3    4    5    6    7    8    9   10
```

NO   MODERATE   WORST

PAIN   PAIN   POSSIBLE

1. What is your current level of pain? (Use chart above) _____
2. What level do you want your pain level to be at? _____
3. What is the worst pain level you can handle? _____
4. Where do you want to improve the most?

   _____

5. Regarding Question #2, Why?

   _____

   _____

6. What are you currently doing to treat your pain? (List all treatments)

   _____

   _____

7. What would you like to add to your regimen to try and control your condition? (Medications, Exercise, Medical Devices, etc.)

   _____

   _____

8. How many "Quality" hours of sleep do you get a night?

   _____

9. What do you consider quality sleep? _____

   _____

10. How many time during the night do you wake up? _____
11. Why are you waking up? (Dreams, Pain, Rest Room, Kids, Pets)

   _____

12. How often in a week do you exercise? _____
13. What types of exercise are you doing? For how long? (List all forms)

   _____

14. Is there anything currently that you do which you believe benefits your pain? _____

   _____

   _____

WHAT ARE YOUR CURRENT & LONG TERM GOALS?

(CONTINUED)

15. Are you working? YES / NO, if yes, what do you do? How many days a week do you work? (Provide Details):

_____

_____

16. Are you able to care for yourself or do you have someone who assists you? _____

_____

17. If yes to #18, what areas of your life do they assist you're with?

_____

_____

_____

18. Do you have a family member you care for? YES / NO

19. If yes to #20, how much care do they/you provide?

_____

_____

_____

TIP #349 "A person with chronic pain might need to spread the tasks out over a longer period of time. More breaks (even if they are day long breaks) can be very helpful." *

TIP #302 "Cheer your small successes! Did you finally get through to the medical supply company after the 100th try?
Yay! That's progress." *

EXPENSES FOR: _____/_____

                       (MONTH)   (YEAR)

EXPENSE FOR   **DATE**   **MILES**   **AMOUNT**

1. _____
2. _____
3. _____
4. _____
5. _____
6. _____
7. _____
8. _____
9. _____
10. _____
11. _____
12. _____
13. _____
14. _____
15. _____
16. _____
17. _____
18. _____
19. _____
20. _____
21. _____
22. _____
23. _____
24. _____
25. _____
26. _____
27. _____
28. _____
29. _____
30. _____
31. _____
32. _____
33. _____
34. _____
35. _____

                        TOTALS: _____ / _____

EXTRA SPACE FOR NOTES

_____
_____
_____
_____
_____
_____
_____
_____
_____
_____
_____
_____
_____
_____
_____
_____
_____
_____

TIPS FOR THE CALENDAR

- *Use different colored pens or pencils for each doctor. This way with a glance you will know who is on the schedule for the day.*
- *As soon as an appointment is made, enter it into the calendar. Even if the appointment is three months away it's just more time for you to forget it.*
- *If someone else is also involved in going to the appointments update them as soon as possible and meet 1-2 times a month to compare schedules.*
- *Place an "E" next to any appointment if there is an expense involved. This way you ensure to send it in for reimbursement when needed.*
- *On appointment days, put all stops (lunch, pharmacy, etc.) on the calendar so you don't run short on time.*

DAILY CARE LOG

DATE: _____   DAY: SUN MON TUE WED THU FRI SAT

BLOOD PRESSURE: _____   PULSE: _____   WEIGHT: _____

OXYGEN LEVEL: _____ HOURS OF SLEEP: _____ TIMES AWAKE: _____

QUALITY SLEEP: YES / NO (CIRCLE ONE)   CURRENT PAIN: _____

NEXT APPOINTMENT (DATE, TIME, ETC: _____

IF NOT QUALITY, WHY? _____

MEDICATION TIMES: ____A/P ___A/P ___A/P ___A/P ___A/P ___A/P

OTHER EVENTS / EPISODES: _____
_____
_____

OTHER INFORMATION:
_____
_____

APPOINTMENT WITH: _____ DATE/TIME: _____/_____

REASON FOR VISIT: _____

RESULTS:
_____
_____
_____

NEXT APPOINTMENT (DATE, TIME, ETC): _____

APPOINTMENT WITH: _____ DATE/TIME: _____/_____

REASON FOR VISIT: _____

RESULTS:
_____
_____
_____

MISC..NOTES:
_____
_____
_____

DAILY CARE LOG

DATE: _____   DAY: SUN MON TUE WED THU FRI SAT

BLOOD PRESSURE: _____   PULSE: _____   WEIGHT: _____

OXYGEN LEVEL: _____ HOURS OF SLEEP: _____ TIMES AWAKE: _____

QUALITY SLEEP: YES / NO (CIRCLE ONE)   CURRENT PAIN: _____

NEXT APPOINTMENT (DATE, TIME, ETC: _____

IF NOT QUALITY, WHY? _____

MEDICATION TIMES: ___A/P ___A/P ___A/P ___A/P ___A/P ___A/P

OTHER EVENTS / EPISODES: _____
_____
_____

OTHER INFORMATION:
_____
_____

APPOINTMENT WITH: _____ DATE/TIME: _____/_____

REASON FOR VISIT:
_____

RESULTS:
_____
_____
_____

NEXT APPOINTMENT (DATE, TIME, ETC): _____

APPOINTMENT WITH: _____ DATE/TIME: _____/_____

REASON FOR VISIT:
_____

RESULTS:
_____
_____
_____

MISC..NOTES:
_____
_____
_____

DAILY CARE LOG

DATE: _____   DAY: SUN MON TUE WED THU FRI SAT

BLOOD PRESSURE: _____   PULSE: _____   WEIGHT: _____

OXYGEN LEVEL: _____ HOURS OF SLEEP: _____ TIMES AWAKE: _____

QUALITY SLEEP: YES / NO (CIRCLE ONE)   CURRENT PAIN: _____

NEXT APPOINTMENT (DATE, TIME, ETC: _____

IF NOT QUALITY, WHY? _____

MEDICATION TIMES: ____A/P ___A/P ___A/P ___A/P ___A/P ___A/P

OTHER EVENTS / EPISODES: _____
_____
_____

OTHER INFORMATION:
_____
_____

APPOINTMENT WITH: _____ DATE/TIME: _____/_____

REASON FOR VISIT: _____

RESULTS:
_____
_____
_____

NEXT APPOINTMENT (DATE, TIME, ETC): _____

APPOINTMENT WITH: _____ DATE/TIME: _____/_____

REASON FOR VISIT: _____

RESULTS:
_____
_____
_____

MISC..NOTES:
_____
_____
_____

DAILY CARE LOG

DATE: _____   DAY: SUN MON TUE WED THU FRI SAT

BLOOD PRESSURE: _____ PULSE: _____ WEIGHT: _____

OXYGEN LEVEL: _____ HOURS OF SLEEP: _____ TIMES AWAKE: _____

QUALITY SLEEP: YES / NO (CIRCLE ONE)   CURRENT PAIN: _____

NEXT APPOINTMENT (DATE, TIME, ETC: _____

IF NOT QUALITY, WHY? _____

MEDICATION TIMES: ____A/P ___A/P ___A/P ___A/P ___A/P ___A/P

OTHER EVENTS / EPISODES: _____
_____
_____

OTHER INFORMATION:
_____
_____

APPOINTMENT WITH: _____ DATE/TIME: _____/_____
REASON FOR VISIT:
_____

RESULTS:
_____
_____
_____

NEXT APPOINTMENT (DATE, TIME, ETC): _____
APPOINTMENT WITH: _____ DATE/TIME: _____/_____
REASON FOR VISIT:
_____

RESULTS:
_____
_____
_____

MISC..NOTES:
_____
_____
_____

DAILY CARE LOG

DATE: _____   DAY: SUN MON TUE WED THU FRI SAT

BLOOD PRESSURE: _____   PULSE: _____   WEIGHT: _____

OXYGEN LEVEL: _____ HOURS OF SLEEP: _____ TIMES AWAKE: _____

QUALITY SLEEP: YES / NO (CIRCLE ONE)   CURRENT PAIN: _____

NEXT APPOINTMENT (DATE, TIME, ETC: _____

IF NOT QUALITY, WHY? _____

MEDICATION TIMES: ___A/P ___A/P ___A/P ___A/P ___A/P ___A/P

OTHER EVENTS / EPISODES: _____
_____
_____

OTHER INFORMATION:
_____
_____

APPOINTMENT WITH: _____ DATE/TIME: _____/_____
REASON FOR VISIT: _____
RESULTS:
_____
_____
_____

NEXT APPOINTMENT (DATE, TIME, ETC): _____
APPOINTMENT WITH: _____ DATE/TIME: _____/_____
REASON FOR VISIT: _____
RESULTS:
_____
_____
_____

MISC..NOTES:
_____
_____
_____

DAILY CARE LOG

DATE: _____   DAY: SUN MON TUE WED THU FRI SAT

BLOOD PRESSURE: _____   PULSE: _____   WEIGHT: _____

OXYGEN LEVEL: _____ HOURS OF SLEEP: _____ TIMES AWAKE: _____

QUALITY SLEEP: YES / NO (CIRCLE ONE)   CURRENT PAIN: _____

NEXT APPOINTMENT (DATE, TIME, ETC: _____

IF NOT QUALITY, WHY? _____

MEDICATION TIMES: ____A/P ___A/P ____A/P ____A/P ____A/P ____A/P

OTHER EVENTS / EPISODES: _____
_____
_____

OTHER INFORMATION:
_____
_____

APPOINTMENT WITH: _____ DATE/TIME: _____/_____
REASON FOR VISIT:
_____

RESULTS:
_____
_____
_____

NEXT APPOINTMENT (DATE, TIME, ETC): _____
APPOINTMENT WITH: _____ DATE/TIME: _____/_____
REASON FOR VISIT:
_____

RESULTS:
_____
_____
_____

MISC..NOTES:
_____
_____
_____

DAILY CARE LOG

DATE: _____   DAY: SUN MON TUE WED THU FRI SAT

BLOOD PRESSURE: _____   PULSE: _____   WEIGHT: _____

OXYGEN LEVEL: _____ HOURS OF SLEEP: _____ TIMES AWAKE: _____

QUALITY SLEEP: YES / NO (CIRCLE ONE)   CURRENT PAIN: _____

NEXT APPOINTMENT (DATE, TIME, ETC: _____

IF NOT QUALITY, WHY? _____

MEDICATION TIMES: ____A/P ___A/P ___A/P ___A/P ___A/P ___A/P

OTHER EVENTS / EPISODES: _____
_____
_____

OTHER INFORMATION:
_____
_____

APPOINTMENT WITH: _____ DATE/TIME: _____/_____

REASON FOR VISIT: _____

RESULTS:
_____
_____
_____

NEXT APPOINTMENT (DATE, TIME, ETC): _____

APPOINTMENT WITH: _____ DATE/TIME: _____/_____

REASON FOR VISIT: _____

RESULTS:
_____
_____
_____

MISC..NOTES:
_____
_____
_____

DAILY CARE LOG

DATE: _____   DAY: SUN MON TUE WED THU FRI SAT

BLOOD PRESSURE: _____   PULSE: _____   WEIGHT: _____

OXYGEN LEVEL: _____ HOURS OF SLEEP: _____ TIMES AWAKE: _____

QUALITY SLEEP: YES / NO (CIRCLE ONE)   CURRENT PAIN: _____

NEXT APPOINTMENT (DATE, TIME, ETC: _____

IF NOT QUALITY, WHY? _____

MEDICATION TIMES: ____A/P ____A/P ____A/P ____A/P ____A/P ____A/P

OTHER EVENTS / EPISODES: _____
_____
_____

OTHER INFORMATION:
_____
_____

APPOINTMENT WITH: _____ DATE/TIME: _____/_____
REASON FOR VISIT:
_____

RESULTS:
_____
_____
_____

NEXT APPOINTMENT (DATE, TIME, ETC): _____
APPOINTMENT WITH: _____ DATE/TIME: _____/_____
REASON FOR VISIT:
_____

RESULTS:
_____
_____
_____

MISC..NOTES:
_____
_____
_____

DAILY CARE LOG

DATE: _____   DAY: SUN MON TUE WED THU FRI SAT

BLOOD PRESSURE: _____   PULSE: _____   WEIGHT: _____

OXYGEN LEVEL: _____ HOURS OF SLEEP: _____ TIMES AWAKE: _____

QUALITY SLEEP: YES / NO (CIRCLE ONE)   CURRENT PAIN: _____

NEXT APPOINTMENT (DATE, TIME, ETC: _____

IF NOT QUALITY, WHY? _____

MEDICATION TIMES: ____A/P ___A/P ___A/P ___A/P ___A/P ___A/P

OTHER EVENTS / EPISODES: _____
_____
_____

OTHER INFORMATION:
_____
_____

APPOINTMENT WITH: _____ DATE/TIME: _____/_____
REASON FOR VISIT: _____
RESULTS:
_____
_____
_____

NEXT APPOINTMENT (DATE, TIME, ETC): _____
APPOINTMENT WITH: _____ DATE/TIME: _____/_____
REASON FOR VISIT: _____
RESULTS:
_____
_____
_____

MISC..NOTES:
_____
_____
_____

DAILY CARE LOG

DATE: _____   DAY: SUN MON TUE WED THU FRI SAT

BLOOD PRESSURE: _____   PULSE: _____   WEIGHT: _____

OXYGEN LEVEL: _____ HOURS OF SLEEP: _____ TIMES AWAKE: _____

QUALITY SLEEP: YES / NO (CIRCLE ONE)   CURRENT PAIN: _____

NEXT APPOINTMENT (DATE, TIME, ETC: _____

IF NOT QUALITY, WHY? _____

MEDICATION TIMES: ___A/P ___A/P ___A/P ___A/P ___A/P ___A/P

OTHER EVENTS / EPISODES: _____
_____
_____

OTHER INFORMATION:
_____
_____

APPOINTMENT WITH: _____ DATE/TIME: _____/_____

REASON FOR VISIT:
_____

RESULTS:
_____
_____
_____

NEXT APPOINTMENT (DATE, TIME, ETC): _____

APPOINTMENT WITH: _____ DATE/TIME: _____/_____

REASON FOR VISIT:
_____

RESULTS:
_____
_____
_____

MISC..NOTES:
_____
_____
_____

DAILY CARE LOG

DATE: _____ DAY: SUN MON TUE WED THU FRI SAT

BLOOD PRESSURE: _____ PULSE: _____ WEIGHT: _____

OXYGEN LEVEL: _____ HOURS OF SLEEP: _____ TIMES AWAKE: _____

QUALITY SLEEP: YES / NO (CIRCLE ONE) CURRENT PAIN: _____

NEXT APPOINTMENT (DATE, TIME, ETC: _____

IF NOT QUALITY, WHY? _____

MEDICATION TIMES: ____A/P ___A/P ___A/P ___A/P ___A/P ___A/P

OTHER EVENTS / EPISODES: _____
_____
_____

OTHER INFORMATION:
_____
_____

APPOINTMENT WITH: _____ DATE/TIME: _____/_____
REASON FOR VISIT: _____
RESULTS:
_____
_____
_____

NEXT APPOINTMENT (DATE, TIME, ETC): _____
APPOINTMENT WITH: _____ DATE/TIME: _____/_____
REASON FOR VISIT: _____
RESULTS:
_____
_____
_____

MISC..NOTES:
_____
_____
_____

DAILY CARE LOG

DATE: _____   DAY: SUN MON TUE WED THU FRI SAT

BLOOD PRESSURE: _____   PULSE: _____   WEIGHT: _____

OXYGEN LEVEL: _____ HOURS OF SLEEP: _____ TIMES AWAKE: _____

QUALITY SLEEP: YES / NO (CIRCLE ONE)   CURRENT PAIN: _____

NEXT APPOINTMENT (DATE, TIME, ETC: _____

IF NOT QUALITY, WHY? _____

MEDICATION TIMES: ____A/P ____A/P ____A/P ____A/P ____A/P ____A/P

OTHER EVENTS / EPISODES: _____
_____
_____

OTHER INFORMATION:
_____
_____

APPOINTMENT WITH: _____ DATE/TIME: _____/_____
REASON FOR VISIT:
_____

RESULTS:
_____
_____
_____

NEXT APPOINTMENT (DATE, TIME, ETC): _____
APPOINTMENT WITH: _____ DATE/TIME: _____/_____
REASON FOR VISIT:
_____

RESULTS:
_____
_____
_____

MISC..NOTES:
_____
_____
_____

DAILY CARE LOG

DATE: _____   DAY: SUN MON TUE WED THU FRI SAT

BLOOD PRESSURE: _____   PULSE: _____   WEIGHT: _____

OXYGEN LEVEL: _____ HOURS OF SLEEP: _____ TIMES AWAKE: _____

QUALITY SLEEP: YES / NO (CIRCLE ONE)   CURRENT PAIN: _____

NEXT APPOINTMENT (DATE, TIME, ETC: _____

IF NOT QUALITY, WHY? _____

MEDICATION TIMES: ____A/P ___A/P ___A/P ___A/P ___A/P ___A/P

OTHER EVENTS / EPISODES: _____
_____
_____

OTHER INFORMATION:
_____
_____

APPOINTMENT WITH: _____ DATE/TIME: _____/_____

REASON FOR VISIT: _____

RESULTS:
_____
_____
_____

NEXT APPOINTMENT (DATE, TIME, ETC): _____

APPOINTMENT WITH: _____ DATE/TIME: _____/_____

REASON FOR VISIT: _____

RESULTS:
_____
_____
_____

MISC..NOTES:
_____
_____
_____

DAILY CARE LOG

DATE: _____   DAY: SUN MON TUE WED THU FRI SAT

BLOOD PRESSURE: _____   PULSE: _____   WEIGHT: _____

OXYGEN LEVEL: _____ HOURS OF SLEEP: _____ TIMES AWAKE: _____

QUALITY SLEEP: YES / NO (CIRCLE ONE)   CURRENT PAIN: _____

NEXT APPOINTMENT (DATE, TIME, ETC: _____

IF NOT QUALITY, WHY? _____

MEDICATION TIMES: ____A/P ___A/P ___A/P ___A/P ___A/P ___A/P

OTHER EVENTS / EPISODES: _____
_____
_____

OTHER INFORMATION:
_____
_____

APPOINTMENT WITH: _____ DATE/TIME: _____/_____

REASON FOR VISIT:
_____

RESULTS:
_____
_____
_____

NEXT APPOINTMENT (DATE, TIME, ETC): _____

APPOINTMENT WITH: _____ DATE/TIME: _____/_____

REASON FOR VISIT:
_____

RESULTS:
_____
_____
_____

MISC..NOTES:
_____
_____
_____

<u>DAILY CARE LOG</u>

DATE: _____   DAY: SUN MON TUE WED THU FRI SAT

BLOOD PRESSURE: _____   PULSE: _____   WEIGHT: _____

OXYGEN LEVEL: _____ HOURS OF SLEEP: _____ TIMES AWAKE: _____

QUALITY SLEEP: YES / NO (CIRCLE ONE)   CURRENT PAIN: _____

NEXT APPOINTMENT (DATE, TIME, ETC: _____

IF NOT QUALITY, WHY? _____

MEDICATION TIMES: ____A/P ___A/P ___A/P ___A/P ___A/P ___A/P

OTHER EVENTS / EPISODES: _____
_____
_____

OTHER INFORMATION:
_____
_____

APPOINTMENT WITH: _____ DATE/TIME: _____/ _____
REASON FOR VISIT: _____
RESULTS:
_____
_____
_____

NEXT APPOINTMENT (DATE, TIME, ETC): _____
APPOINTMENT WITH: _____ DATE/TIME: _____/ _____
REASON FOR VISIT: _____
RESULTS:
_____
_____
_____

MISC..NOTES:
_____
_____
_____

DAILY CARE LOG

DATE: _____   DAY: SUN MON TUE WED THU FRI SAT

BLOOD PRESSURE: _____   PULSE: _____   WEIGHT: _____

OXYGEN LEVEL: _____ HOURS OF SLEEP: _____ TIMES AWAKE: _____

QUALITY SLEEP: YES / NO (CIRCLE ONE)   CURRENT PAIN: _____

NEXT APPOINTMENT (DATE, TIME, ETC: _____

IF NOT QUALITY, WHY? _____

MEDICATION TIMES: ____A/P ___A/P ___A/P ___A/P ___A/P ___A/P

OTHER EVENTS / EPISODES: _____
_____
_____

OTHER INFORMATION:
_____
_____

APPOINTMENT WITH: _____ DATE/TIME: _____/_____
REASON FOR VISIT:
_____

RESULTS:
_____
_____
_____

NEXT APPOINTMENT (DATE, TIME, ETC): _____
APPOINTMENT WITH: _____ DATE/TIME: _____/_____
REASON FOR VISIT:
_____

RESULTS:
_____
_____
_____

MISC..NOTES:
_____
_____
_____

DAILY CARE LOG

DATE: _____ DAY: SUN MON TUE WED THU FRI SAT

BLOOD PRESSURE: _____ PULSE: _____ WEIGHT: _____

OXYGEN LEVEL: _____ HOURS OF SLEEP: _____ TIMES AWAKE: _____

QUALITY SLEEP: YES / NO (CIRCLE ONE)   CURRENT PAIN: _____

NEXT APPOINTMENT (DATE, TIME, ETC: _____

IF NOT QUALITY, WHY? _____

MEDICATION TIMES: ____A/P ___A/P ___A/P ___A/P ___A/P ___A/P

OTHER EVENTS / EPISODES: _____
_____
_____

OTHER INFORMATION:
_____
_____

APPOINTMENT WITH: _____ DATE/TIME: _____/_____

REASON FOR VISIT: _____

RESULTS:
_____
_____
_____

NEXT APPOINTMENT (DATE, TIME, ETC): _____

APPOINTMENT WITH: _____ DATE/TIME: _____/_____

REASON FOR VISIT: _____

RESULTS:
_____
_____
_____

MISC..NOTES:
_____
_____
_____

DAILY CARE LOG

DATE: _____ DAY: SUN MON TUE WED THU FRI SAT

BLOOD PRESSURE: _____ PULSE: _____ WEIGHT: _____

OXYGEN LEVEL: _____ HOURS OF SLEEP: _____ TIMES AWAKE: _____

QUALITY SLEEP: YES / NO (CIRCLE ONE)   CURRENT PAIN: _____

NEXT APPOINTMENT (DATE, TIME, ETC: _____

IF NOT QUALITY, WHY? _____

MEDICATION TIMES: ____A/P ___A/P ___A/P ___A/P ___A/P ___A/P

OTHER EVENTS / EPISODES: _____
_____
_____

OTHER INFORMATION:
_____
_____

APPOINTMENT WITH: _____ DATE/TIME: _____/_____
REASON FOR VISIT:
_____

RESULTS:
_____
_____
_____

NEXT APPOINTMENT (DATE, TIME, ETC): _____
APPOINTMENT WITH: _____ DATE/TIME: _____/_____
REASON FOR VISIT:
_____

RESULTS:
_____
_____
_____

MISC..NOTES:
_____
_____
_____

DAILY CARE LOG

DATE: _____   DAY: SUN MON TUE WED THU FRI SAT

BLOOD PRESSURE: _____   PULSE: _____   WEIGHT: _____

OXYGEN LEVEL: _____ HOURS OF SLEEP: _____ TIMES AWAKE: _____

QUALITY SLEEP: YES / NO (CIRCLE ONE)   CURRENT PAIN: _____

NEXT APPOINTMENT (DATE, TIME, ETC: _____

IF NOT QUALITY, WHY? _____

MEDICATION TIMES: ____A/P ___A/P ___A/P ___A/P ___A/P ___A/P

OTHER EVENTS / EPISODES: _____
_____
_____

OTHER INFORMATION:
_____
_____

APPOINTMENT WITH: _____ DATE/TIME: _____/ _____

REASON FOR VISIT: _____

RESULTS:
_____
_____
_____

NEXT APPOINTMENT (DATE, TIME, ETC): _____

APPOINTMENT WITH: _____ DATE/TIME: _____/ _____

REASON FOR VISIT: _____

RESULTS:
_____
_____
_____

MISC..NOTES:
_____
_____
_____

DAILY CARE LOG

DATE: _____   DAY: SUN MON TUE WED THU FRI SAT

BLOOD PRESSURE: _____   PULSE: _____   WEIGHT: _____

OXYGEN LEVEL: _____ HOURS OF SLEEP: _____ TIMES AWAKE: _____

QUALITY SLEEP: YES / NO (CIRCLE ONE)   CURRENT PAIN: _____

NEXT APPOINTMENT (DATE, TIME, ETC: _____

IF NOT QUALITY, WHY? _____

MEDICATION TIMES: ____A/P ___A/P ____A/P ____A/P ____A/P ____A/P

OTHER EVENTS / EPISODES: _____
_____
_____

OTHER INFORMATION:
_____
_____

APPOINTMENT WITH: _____ DATE/TIME: _____/_____

REASON FOR VISIT:
_____

RESULTS:
_____
_____
_____

NEXT APPOINTMENT (DATE, TIME, ETC): _____

APPOINTMENT WITH: _____ DATE/TIME: _____/_____

REASON FOR VISIT:
_____

RESULTS:
_____
_____
_____

MISC..NOTES:
_____
_____
_____

DAILY CARE LOG

DATE: _____   DAY: SUN MON TUE WED THU FRI SAT

BLOOD PRESSURE: _____   PULSE: _____   WEIGHT: _____

OXYGEN LEVEL: _____ HOURS OF SLEEP: _____ TIMES AWAKE: _____

QUALITY SLEEP: YES / NO (CIRCLE ONE)   CURRENT PAIN: _____

NEXT APPOINTMENT (DATE, TIME, ETC: _____

IF NOT QUALITY, WHY? _____

MEDICATION TIMES: ____A/P ___A/P ___A/P ____A/P ___A/P ___A/P

OTHER EVENTS / EPISODES: _____
_____
_____

OTHER INFORMATION:
_____
_____

APPOINTMENT WITH: _____ DATE/TIME: _____/_____

REASON FOR VISIT: _____

RESULTS:
_____
_____
_____

NEXT APPOINTMENT (DATE, TIME, ETC): _____

APPOINTMENT WITH: _____ DATE/TIME: _____/_____

REASON FOR VISIT: _____

RESULTS:
_____
_____
_____

MISC..NOTES:
_____
_____
_____

DAILY CARE LOG

DATE: _____   DAY: SUN MON TUE WED THU FRI SAT

BLOOD PRESSURE: _____   PULSE: _____   WEIGHT: _____

OXYGEN LEVEL: _____ HOURS OF SLEEP: _____ TIMES AWAKE: _____

QUALITY SLEEP: YES / NO (CIRCLE ONE)   CURRENT PAIN: _____

NEXT APPOINTMENT (DATE, TIME, ETC: _____

IF NOT QUALITY, WHY? _____

MEDICATION TIMES: ____A/P ___A/P ___A/P ___A/P ___A/P ___A/P

OTHER EVENTS / EPISODES: _____
_____
_____

OTHER INFORMATION:
_____
_____

APPOINTMENT WITH: _____ DATE/TIME: _____/_____

REASON FOR VISIT:
_____

RESULTS:
_____
_____
_____

NEXT APPOINTMENT (DATE, TIME, ETC): _____

APPOINTMENT WITH: _____ DATE/TIME: _____/_____

REASON FOR VISIT:
_____

RESULTS:
_____
_____
_____

MISC..NOTES:
_____
_____
_____

DAILY CARE LOG

DATE: _____   DAY: SUN MON TUE WED THU FRI SAT

BLOOD PRESSURE: _____   PULSE: _____   WEIGHT: _____

OXYGEN LEVEL: _____ HOURS OF SLEEP: _____ TIMES AWAKE: _____

QUALITY SLEEP: YES / NO (CIRCLE ONE)   CURRENT PAIN: _____

NEXT APPOINTMENT (DATE, TIME, ETC: _____

IF NOT QUALITY, WHY? _____

MEDICATION TIMES: ____A/P ___A/P ___A/P ___A/P ___A/P ___A/P

OTHER EVENTS / EPISODES: _____
_____
_____

OTHER INFORMATION:
_____
_____

APPOINTMENT WITH: _____ DATE/TIME: _____/_____
REASON FOR VISIT: _____
RESULTS:
_____
_____
_____

NEXT APPOINTMENT (DATE, TIME, ETC): _____
APPOINTMENT WITH: _____ DATE/TIME: _____/_____
REASON FOR VISIT: _____
RESULTS:
_____
_____
_____

MISC..NOTES:
_____
_____
_____

DAILY CARE LOG

DATE: _____   DAY: SUN MON TUE WED THU FRI SAT

BLOOD PRESSURE: _____   PULSE: _____   WEIGHT: _____

OXYGEN LEVEL: _____ HOURS OF SLEEP: _____ TIMES AWAKE: _____

QUALITY SLEEP: YES / NO (CIRCLE ONE)   CURRENT PAIN: _____

NEXT APPOINTMENT (DATE, TIME, ETC: _____

IF NOT QUALITY, WHY? _____

MEDICATION TIMES: ____A/P ___A/P ___A/P ___A/P ___A/P ___A/P

OTHER EVENTS / EPISODES: _____
_____
_____

OTHER INFORMATION:
_____
_____

APPOINTMENT WITH: _____ DATE/TIME: _____/_____

REASON FOR VISIT:
_____

RESULTS:
_____
_____
_____

NEXT APPOINTMENT (DATE, TIME, ETC): _____

APPOINTMENT WITH: _____ DATE/TIME: _____/_____

REASON FOR VISIT:
_____

RESULTS:
_____
_____
_____

MISC..NOTES:
_____
_____
_____

DAILY CARE LOG

DATE: _____   DAY: SUN MON TUE WED THU FRI SAT

BLOOD PRESSURE: _____   PULSE: _____   WEIGHT: _____

OXYGEN LEVEL: _____ HOURS OF SLEEP: _____ TIMES AWAKE: _____

QUALITY SLEEP: YES / NO (CIRCLE ONE)   CURRENT PAIN: _____

NEXT APPOINTMENT (DATE, TIME, ETC: _____

IF NOT QUALITY, WHY? _____

MEDICATION TIMES: ____A/P ___A/P ___A/P ___A/P ___A/P ___A/P

OTHER EVENTS / EPISODES: _____
_____
_____

OTHER INFORMATION:
_____
_____

APPOINTMENT WITH: _____ DATE/TIME: _____/ _____

REASON FOR VISIT: _____

RESULTS:
_____
_____
_____

NEXT APPOINTMENT (DATE, TIME, ETC): _____

APPOINTMENT WITH: _____ DATE/TIME: _____/ _____

REASON FOR VISIT: _____

RESULTS:
_____
_____
_____

MISC..NOTES:
_____
_____
_____

DAILY CARE LOG

DATE: _____   DAY: SUN MON TUE WED THU FRI SAT

BLOOD PRESSURE: _____   PULSE: _____   WEIGHT: _____

OXYGEN LEVEL: _____ HOURS OF SLEEP: _____ TIMES AWAKE: _____

QUALITY SLEEP: YES / NO (CIRCLE ONE)   CURRENT PAIN: _____

NEXT APPOINTMENT (DATE, TIME, ETC: _____

IF NOT QUALITY, WHY? _____

MEDICATION TIMES: ____A/P ___A/P ___A/P ___A/P ___A/P ___A/P

OTHER EVENTS / EPISODES: _____
_____
_____

OTHER INFORMATION:
_____
_____

APPOINTMENT WITH: _____ DATE/TIME: _____/_____
REASON FOR VISIT:
_____

RESULTS:
_____
_____
_____

NEXT APPOINTMENT (DATE, TIME, ETC): _____
APPOINTMENT WITH: _____ DATE/TIME: _____/_____
REASON FOR VISIT:
_____

RESULTS:
_____
_____
_____

MISC..NOTES:
_____
_____
_____

DAILY CARE LOG

DATE: _____   DAY: SUN MON TUE WED THU FRI SAT

BLOOD PRESSURE: _____   PULSE: _____   WEIGHT: _____

OXYGEN LEVEL: _____ HOURS OF SLEEP: _____ TIMES AWAKE: _____

QUALITY SLEEP: YES / NO (CIRCLE ONE)   CURRENT PAIN: _____

NEXT APPOINTMENT (DATE, TIME, ETC: _____

IF NOT QUALITY, WHY? _____

MEDICATION TIMES: ____A/P ___A/P ___A/P ___A/P ___A/P ___A/P

OTHER EVENTS / EPISODES: _____
_____
_____

OTHER INFORMATION:
_____
_____

APPOINTMENT WITH: _____ DATE/TIME: _____/ _____
REASON FOR VISIT: _____
RESULTS:
_____
_____
_____

NEXT APPOINTMENT (DATE, TIME, ETC): _____
APPOINTMENT WITH: _____ DATE/TIME: _____/ _____
REASON FOR VISIT: _____
RESULTS:
_____
_____
_____

MISC..NOTES:
_____
_____
_____

DAILY CARE LOG

DATE: _____   DAY: SUN MON TUE WED THU FRI SAT

BLOOD PRESSURE: _____   PULSE: _____   WEIGHT: _____

OXYGEN LEVEL: _____ HOURS OF SLEEP: _____ TIMES AWAKE: _____

QUALITY SLEEP: YES / NO (CIRCLE ONE)   CURRENT PAIN: _____

NEXT APPOINTMENT (DATE, TIME, ETC: _____

IF NOT QUALITY, WHY? _____

MEDICATION TIMES: ____A/P ___A/P ___A/P ___A/P ___A/P ___A/P

OTHER EVENTS / EPISODES: _____
_____
_____

OTHER INFORMATION:
_____
_____

APPOINTMENT WITH: _____ DATE/TIME: _____/_____
REASON FOR VISIT:
_____

RESULTS:
_____
_____
_____

NEXT APPOINTMENT (DATE, TIME, ETC): _____
APPOINTMENT WITH: _____ DATE/TIME: _____/_____
REASON FOR VISIT:
_____

RESULTS:
_____
_____
_____

MISC..NOTES:
_____
_____
_____

DAILY CARE LOG

DATE: _____ DAY: SUN MON TUE WED THU FRI SAT

BLOOD PRESSURE: _____ PULSE: _____ WEIGHT: _____

OXYGEN LEVEL: _____ HOURS OF SLEEP: _____ TIMES AWAKE: _____

QUALITY SLEEP: YES / NO (CIRCLE ONE) CURRENT PAIN: _____

NEXT APPOINTMENT (DATE, TIME, ETC: _____

IF NOT QUALITY, WHY? _____

MEDICATION TIMES: ___A/P ___A/P ___A/P ___A/P ___A/P ___A/P

OTHER EVENTS / EPISODES: _____
_____
_____

OTHER INFORMATION:
_____
_____

APPOINTMENT WITH: _____ DATE/TIME: _____/_____

REASON FOR VISIT: _____

RESULTS:
_____
_____
_____

NEXT APPOINTMENT (DATE, TIME, ETC): _____

APPOINTMENT WITH: _____ DATE/TIME: _____/_____

REASON FOR VISIT: _____

RESULTS:
_____
_____
_____

MISC..NOTES:
_____
_____
_____

DAILY CARE LOG

DATE: _____   DAY: SUN MON TUE WED THU FRI SAT

BLOOD PRESSURE: _____ PULSE: _____ WEIGHT: _____

OXYGEN LEVEL: _____ HOURS OF SLEEP: _____ TIMES AWAKE: _____

QUALITY SLEEP: YES / NO (CIRCLE ONE)   CURRENT PAIN: _____

NEXT APPOINTMENT (DATE, TIME, ETC: _____

IF NOT QUALITY, WHY? _____

MEDICATION TIMES: ____A/P ___A/P ____A/P ___A/P ___A/P ___A/P

OTHER EVENTS / EPISODES: _____
_____
_____

OTHER INFORMATION:
_____
_____

APPOINTMENT WITH: _____ DATE/TIME: _____/_____

REASON FOR VISIT:
_____

RESULTS:
_____
_____
_____

NEXT APPOINTMENT (DATE, TIME, ETC): _____

APPOINTMENT WITH: _____ DATE/TIME: _____/_____

REASON FOR VISIT:
_____

RESULTS:
_____
_____
_____

MISC..NOTES:
_____
_____
_____

DAILY CARE LOG

DATE: _____   DAY: SUN MON TUE WED THU FRI SAT

BLOOD PRESSURE: _____ PULSE: _____ WEIGHT: _____

OXYGEN LEVEL: _____ HOURS OF SLEEP: _____ TIMES AWAKE: _____

QUALITY SLEEP: YES / NO (CIRCLE ONE)   CURRENT PAIN: _____

NEXT APPOINTMENT (DATE, TIME, ETC: _____

IF NOT QUALITY, WHY? _____

MEDICATION TIMES: ___A/P ___A/P ___A/P ___A/P ___A/P ___A/P

OTHER EVENTS / EPISODES: _____
_____
_____

OTHER INFORMATION: _____
_____
_____

APPOINTMENT WITH: _____ DATE/TIME: _____/_____
REASON FOR VISIT: _____
RESULTS: _____
_____
_____

NEXT APPOINTMENT (DATE, TIME, ETC): _____
APPOINTMENT WITH: _____ DATE/TIME: _____/_____
REASON FOR VISIT: _____
RESULTS: _____
_____
_____

MISC..NOTES: _____
_____
_____

DAILY CARE LOG

DATE: _____   DAY: SUN MON TUE WED THU FRI SAT

BLOOD PRESSURE: _____   PULSE: _____   WEIGHT: _____

OXYGEN LEVEL: _____ HOURS OF SLEEP: _____ TIMES AWAKE: _____

QUALITY SLEEP: YES / NO (CIRCLE ONE)   CURRENT PAIN: _____

NEXT APPOINTMENT (DATE, TIME, ETC: _____

IF NOT QUALITY, WHY? _____

MEDICATION TIMES: ____A/P ___A/P ___A/P ___A/P ___A/P ___A/P

OTHER EVENTS / EPISODES: _____
_____
_____

OTHER INFORMATION:
_____
_____

APPOINTMENT WITH: _____ DATE/TIME: _____/_____

REASON FOR VISIT:
_____

RESULTS:
_____
_____
_____

NEXT APPOINTMENT (DATE, TIME, ETC): _____

APPOINTMENT WITH: _____ DATE/TIME: _____/_____

REASON FOR VISIT:
_____

RESULTS:
_____
_____
_____

MISC..NOTES:
_____
_____
_____

DAILY CARE LOG

DATE: _____ DAY: SUN MON TUE WED THU FRI SAT

BLOOD PRESSURE: _____ PULSE: _____ WEIGHT: _____

OXYGEN LEVEL: _____ HOURS OF SLEEP: _____ TIMES AWAKE: _____

QUALITY SLEEP: YES / NO (CIRCLE ONE) CURRENT PAIN: _____

NEXT APPOINTMENT (DATE, TIME, ETC: _____

IF NOT QUALITY, WHY? _____

MEDICATION TIMES: ____A/P ___A/P ___A/P ___A/P ___A/P ___A/P

OTHER EVENTS / EPISODES: _____
_____
_____

OTHER INFORMATION:
_____
_____

APPOINTMENT WITH: _____ DATE/TIME: _____/_____
REASON FOR VISIT: _____
RESULTS:
_____
_____
_____

NEXT APPOINTMENT (DATE, TIME, ETC): _____
APPOINTMENT WITH: _____ DATE/TIME: _____/_____
REASON FOR VISIT: _____
RESULTS:
_____
_____
_____

MISC..NOTES:
_____
_____
_____

SUCCESSES FOR THE MONTH

_____
_____
_____
_____
_____
_____
_____
_____
_____
_____
_____
_____
_____
_____
_____
_____

"The strength is smiling when you want to cry, Laughing
to hide the pain,
And going on no matter what." ~ Unknown

THINGS TO TRY DIFFERENT

_____
_____
_____
_____
_____
_____
_____

THANK YOU!!

Thank you for your purchase of, "A Journal of Care." I hope you were able to use it to its fullest extent. If you found a way to improve on it and make it easier for you or other caregivers going through the same situation, please feel free to let us know and we can easily add "your idea" into the next books being sent out. And on the other end of things, if you found an area to be not so useful for your situation we are happy to hear that also. The designing of this journal is meant to be a "General One" to be used by all medical conditions (Chronic Pain, Alzheimer's, Epilepsy, Fibromyalgia, Dementia, etc.) so it is not a 100% for just one ailment, I would like to start setting them up that way because different ailments monitor and have different side effects that need to be watched.

It is also designed to:
1. Make it as easy as possible for you-the caregiver-to enter the date obtained on you or your loved one.
2. Make it as easy as possible for the medical personnel (technicians, nurses, doctors, pharmacist, etc.) to locate and read the information they need if you're unable to show them.
3. Make it easy for you to carry around when you're having to carry a to-go bag, purse, coffee all while trying to push a wheelchair, ensuring the walkers legs don't go into a pothole or that your loved one doesn't fall over.
4. The size of the journal was important because I've been there. I've pushed mom while carrying bags, meal tray and more the journal had to fit into a purse, backpack or the pocket on the back of a wheelchair, no exception.

Thank you again to everyone for your support and your business. Additional copies of, "A Journal of Care," are available in 1 month, 3 months and 6 month lengths through the supplier where this journal was purchased or send an email to iCareConsulting@att.net.

Thank you all,
Richard Kreis

www.ingramcontent.com/pod-product-compliance
Lightning Source LLC
Chambersburg PA
CBHW050337290526
45785CB00006B/2534